# Good Flow

YOUR HOLISTIC GUIDE TO
THE BEST PERIOD
OF YOUR LIFE

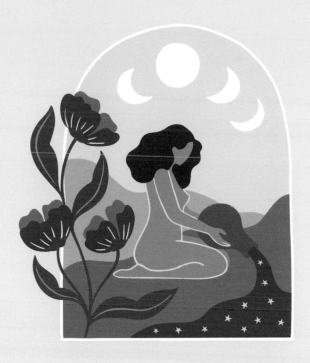

# Good Flow

## YOUR HOLISTIC GUIDE TO
## THE BEST PERIOD OF YOUR LIFE

Julia Blohberger and Roos Neeter

Illustrations by Roel Steenbergen

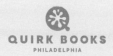

QUIRK BOOKS

PHILADELPHIA

THIS BOOK BELONGS TO:

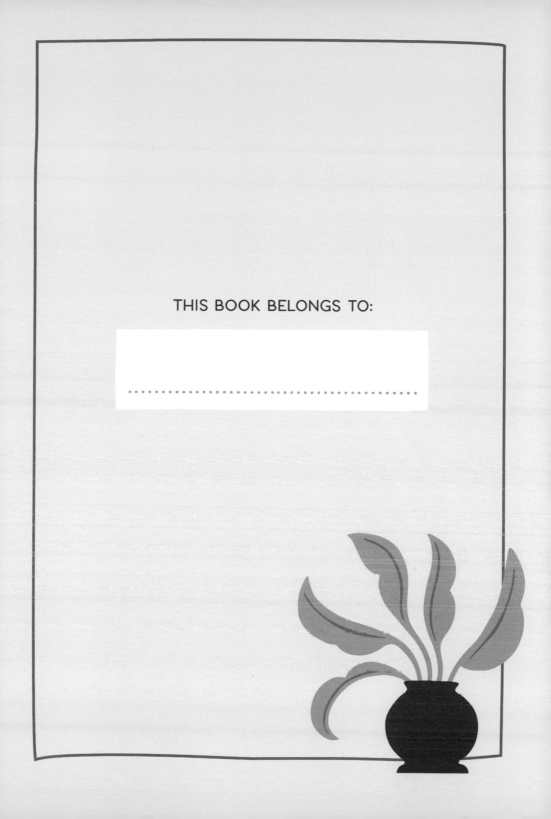

# Contents

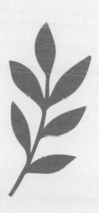

# Get into the Flow

If you have a uterus, chances are you have a period. And if you have a period, chances are you hate it.

Menstruation comes with pain, inconvenience, mess, and emotional upheaval. Even worse, many cultures have shame or stigma about periods. If you've ever canceled a date because of bleeding, hidden a tampon in your hand so people won't know why you're going to the bathroom, gritted your teeth through cramps so you don't have to admit why you're in pain, or used euphemisms like "Aunt Flo" or "that time of the month," you've been affected by cultural attitudes telling you that periods are embarrassing and unmentionable.

As professionally trained and certified Ayurveda instructors, we have a different attitude. We see menstruation as normal, healthy, and worthy of respect. That's why we've put together this guide to help you reconnect with your body's natural cycles, without anxiety or shame. We've included rituals and meditations for checking in with your body, herbal remedies to help with period symptoms, and advice for eating, exercise, journaling, and self-care that accounts for where you are in your cycle.

If you haven't encountered Ayurveda before, don't worry! All you need to know for this book is that we'll be looking at your period *holistically*, as something that affects and is affected by your physical and mental health and everything else going on in your life. We'll be talking about how your body uses and manifests *prana*, or life force, which is analogous to the concept of energy. We'll occasionally use Sanskrit words, because Ayurveda is a practice that originated in India and has deep roots there, but we'll always tell you what they mean for you and for your period.

One thing that makes this book different from other wellness books you've seen before is that we'll talk about the Ayurvedic elements of earth, water, fire, wind, and space. The elements represent different sets of qualities.

* Earth: heaviness, slowness, stability

* Water: flowing, softness, empathy

* Fire: heat, energy, transformation

* Wind: movement, agility, dryness

* Space: subtleness, lightness, imagination

You may have some of these qualities as innate aspects of your constitution, and they can also be affected by your lifestyle and choices. None of the elements are better or worse than others, but sometimes they can get out of balance, which has ramifications for physical and mental health. As we delve into an Ayurvedic understanding of your period, we'll talk about how you can balance and harmonize these elements. (It's important to note that we're *not* doctors, so please get a doctor's input if your periods are consistently troublesome, and don't take our advice over theirs!)

This book is for people with regular periods, irregular periods, heavy or light periods, painful or easy periods. It's for period newbies and period experts. It's even for people who don't have periods at all because of hormonal birth control, pregnancy, hysterectomy, or menopause. (If you don't have a natural cycle, we suggest you use this book by aligning to the cycle of the moon—full moon for ovulation, new moon for menstruation.)

During your menstruating years, your period can take up as much as a quarter of your life—sometimes more. Our aim is to help you make friends with your cycle, so you can feel balanced and empowered all the time, even that one messy week a month. Let's get flowing!

LOVE, JULIA & ROOS

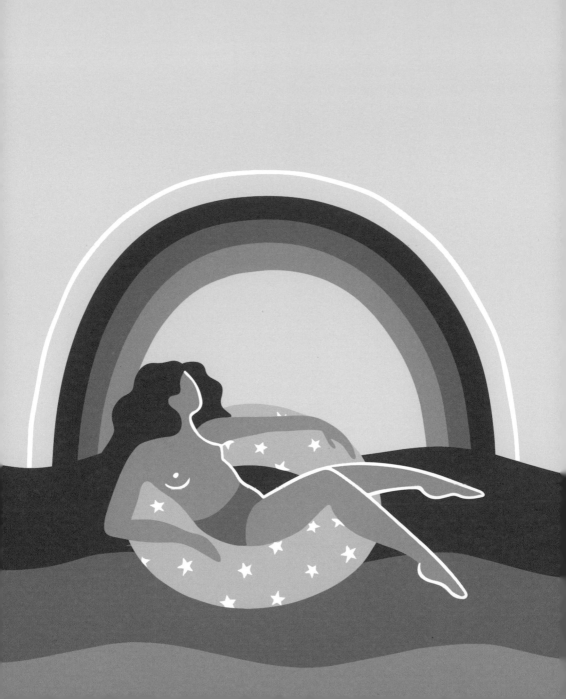

# Periods 101

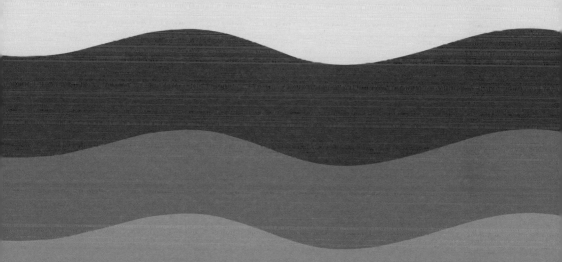

**M**aybe you're new to having a period, or maybe you're an old hand who could use a refresher. Either way, it can be helpful to recap some of the basics of periods, uteruses, and vulvas before we get into anything more complicated.

# The Perfect Cycle

Your period might feel like a monthly burden, but it can also tell you a lot about your health. So let's start by describing the baseline "ideal" period, which indicates that your body is happy and functioning well.

What the perfect cycle looks like will vary from person to person. We all have unique bodies and our individual functioning may vary. Paying attention to the particulars of your period will help you understand what's normal for you. But in general, a normal period will:

* Appear on a regular cycle of twenty-four to thirty-eight days. *Regular* means that it's always about the same amount of time between periods, but this may vary by up to two days in a given cycle.

* Not cause any major discomfort, mentally or physically.

* Produce bright-red blood without a strong smell.

Is this possible? Yes! It's very common to experience pain and discomfort with your period, but it's not inevitable. At the end of this chapter, you'll find a chart to record emotional and physical symptoms of your period. Fill this in during your next cycle to get a snapshot of what your period is like right now. As you implement the techniques from this book, you can use the charts starting on page 112 to observe how your symptoms change over the next few months. (We encourage you to write directly in the book to start, and after that you can photocopy the pages or copy them into a journal or notebook.)

# The Red Rainbow

Menstrual blood is not just blood. It's mixed with tissues from the womb, like cervical fluids and uterine lining. That means it's very normal to see different shades of red during your cycle. But the color of the blood can also indicate health concerns, like problems with circulation or nutrient absorption. Here's what the different colors of blood can tell us about what's going on inside your body.

**Bright red:** This is the color we are looking for. A vibrant red color indicates that you are processing nutrients well. It indicates fresh blood and a steady flow.

**Pink:** Blood that looks a little pinkish can mean that it's mixed with other substances, like cervical fluids. If all of your blood is pink, this might indicate anemia or another problem with how your body processes nutrients.

**Rusty:** You usually see this color at the end of your period. This blood has stayed in the uterus a little longer. When all of your blood has this brownish color, it might mean your blood circulation is not great.

**Purple (and thick):** When blood clots together, the color may look purplish. Small clots are of no concern. If they are very big, you should consult with a doctor.

**Black:** This is a sign of old blood. It can also mean there is a blockage in the vaginal channels.

If you are concerned about the color of your blood please consult with your physician.

# Menstrual Health and Hygiene

Managing your menstrual health and hygiene is fundamental in honoring the cycle. This will prevent infections and other problems in and around your vagina.

*Yoni*, the Sanskrit word for the vagina and vulva, comes from a word meaning "abode." If we look at it from this perspective, you're caring for your yoni the way you would honor and care for your home.

A few things to consider for maximizing health and hygiene during your period:

**Underwear:** You wear underwear right next to your genitals for up to twenty-four hours a day, so you want to make sure these garments aren't exposing you to toxic substances. These days, a lot of underwear is packed with chemicals that are proven to impact hormone levels, so it's better to choose knickers made from organic fabric. Materials you want to look for are organic cotton, organic bamboo, beechwood, organic hemp, and eco-friendly natural dyes.

**Sanitary products:** The method you use to collect blood during your flow can affect the health of your yoni, especially since some period products stay inside your vagina for an extended time. Luckily, there are plenty of suitable options on the market these days. We'll talk more about available products and how to choose among them in the next chapter.

**Wiping:** After a number two, make sure to start with your hand behind yourself and wipe from front to back, away from the vagina. Wiping from the anus toward the vagina is not advised, as it can spread bacteria.

**Washing:** Soap is not necessary. The vagina cleanses itself. Water will do.

# Love Your V

Just like we all have different faces, our vulvas look different too.

It's easy to get caught up in the idea that there's one single way a vulva "should" look—especially since the images of vulvas we encounter may be abstract, as in an anatomy textbook, or airbrushed and idealized, as in porn. But variation in how our genitals look is normal and beautiful! There's no shape, color, or hair situation that's better or worse than others. So let us invite you to fully connect to your vulva as it really looks, without expectation or judgment. Be yourself without shame, embracing the diversity of possible bodies and the uniqueness of where your own vulva falls on that spectrum.

Grab a pen and get in front of a mirror. Draw what you see with love and affection. Celebrating your body can be a gateway into your inherent power.

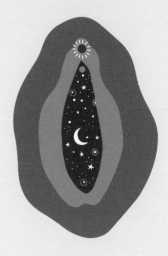

# DRAW YOUR VULVA.

# Welcome to the Pelvic Floor

The pelvic floor is a diamond-shaped group of muscles between your tailbone and your pubic bone. They physically support the bowels and bladder, like a hammock, and they also support the functions of urination, bowel movements, sex, pregnancy, and delivery. Pelvic floor muscles can weaken with age or childbirth, so it's important to give this area plenty of attention to keep it strong and flexible.

To prevent and correct pelvic floor issues, let's start a little higher, with the spine. Have a look at how you sit. Do you sit straight, or in such a way that the spine is rounded and the hips are tilted—in other words, slouching? The spine can be considered the stem of the body, and it is also the location of the main energy channel. Slouching can create blockages in the flow of prana.

At the base of the spine, the psoas muscle extends from the spine through the pelvis. The psoas is a muscle that is very connected to the nervous system. When you're startled or stressed, the psoas contracts as part of your body's fight-or-flight response. An incorrect body posture, and sitting too much in general, will make the psoas weak and stiff. A relaxed psoas will bring calm to the mind.

Other habits that can create a blocked or low flow of prana include:

* Often sitting cross-legged

* Sitting on cold surfaces

* Suppressing natural urges to fart, poop, or pee

* Forcing the same natural urges

* Keeping tension in the pelvis and belly

* Not breathing deeply enough

## WHAT ARE YOUR SITTING HABITS?
## ARE THERE THINGS YOU CAN CHANGE?

# Period Products

These days, there are more period products to choose from than ever! Do you go for a cup or a tampon? Classic sanitary pads or newfangled period underwear? Different options will suit different people, and the most important factor is that you feel safe and comfortable. (We do urge you to choose organic products, especially for anything that's staying inside your vagina.)

**Pads and menstruation underwear:** Sanitary pads are probably the oldest method of period collection—they've been mentioned as far back as the tenth century. You can buy disposable pads, but washable pads made of organic cotton are better for your vaginal health and for the environment. In addition to this well-known approach, there is a new trend: underwear with built-in absorbent padding, which you can wash and reuse. One positive feature of both pads and period underwear is that they do not create any blockage in the passageway of the vagina that can interfere with the natural downward-moving flow.

**Tampons:** A tampon is a piece of absorbent material that sits inside the vagina and soaks up blood. There are two varieties present on the market: one has an integrated applicator, which helps with insertion, and one does not. The applicators are often made of plastic. A more natural approach is to insert the tampon with your fingers; this may take some getting used to, but it reduces waste and also promotes intimacy with your body. A tampon does create a very obvious blockage to the natural downward flow.

**Menstrual cups:** Menstrual cups, flexible cups that sit inside the vagina, have been commercially available since the 1930s, but have increased in popularity in the last few decades. Because they collect blood instead of absorbing it, cups can give you a very clear idea of the amount of blood you are shedding. Another benefit is that you can use the same cup for a longer period of time than a tampon. However, cup use has a learning curve, and if the cup sits crooked or doesn't unfold properly you may find that it starts to leak.

**Free bleeding:** During free bleeding the blood is allowed to flow without being collected. People who free bleed often have activist motivations, like reducing period stigma or protesting the inaccessible cost of period products, but it has other points in its favor. If the idea is appealing to you, we encourage you to do more research—it's too big a topic to get into here!

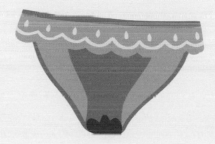

# Spotted!

The main difference between spotting and having your period is the intensity. Spotting is very light, often too light to require period products. Spotting can also happen at any time of the month. A little bit of spotting between periods isn't necessarily a reason for concern. It may even be totally normal. Some of the possible reasons for spotting include:

**Being immediately pre- or post-period:** Often women experience dark-brown spotting just before the onset of the period, or toward the end. This is old blood that has been in contact with oxygen, which is why it looks darker than period blood. If you have dark-brown spotting more than two days before your period begins, consult with your doctor; it can be a sign that your hormone levels are out of balance.

**Ovulation:** Around ovulation you might experience very bright red or pink spotting. This is nothing to worry about—it's due to the natural decline of estrogen at this point in your cycle.

**Implantation:** In some cases, spotting can be an early sign of pregnancy, occurring when the fertilized egg attaches to the endometrium. If you have spotting and you think you might be pregnant, make sure to take a pregnancy test.

**Stress:** Extended periods of stress can affect the hormones. One sign might be that your menstruation becomes very light and irregular, more like spotting. This means the body is too exhausted to produce a healthy flow. That exhaustion can also be caused by overexercising, eating too little, or mental or physical illness.

**Polycystic ovary syndrome (PCOS):** This condition is often accompanied by a lack of ovulation and irregular periods. If you have PCOS, you might sometimes experience only light bleeding or spotting. Make sure to consult with a physician.

## THIS IS YOUR SPACE TO REFLECT ON YOUR RELATIONSHIP WITH YOUR MENSTRUAL CYCLE. IS IT IN BALANCE?

......................................................................................

......................................................................................

......................................................................................

......................................................................................

......................................................................................

......................................................................................

......................................................................................

......................................................................................

......................................................................................

......................................................................................

......................................................................................

......................................................................................

......................................................................................

# WHAT ASPECTS OF YOUR PERIOD
## ARE WORKING FOR YOU?

..........................................................................................................

..........................................................................................................

..........................................................................................................

..........................................................................................................

..........................................................................................................

..........................................................................................................

..........................................................................................................

..........................................................................................................

..........................................................................................................

..........................................................................................................

..........................................................................................................

..........................................................................................................

..........................................................................................................

..........................................................................................................

# WHAT WOULD YOU LIKE TO CHANGE
## ABOUT YOUR PERIOD?

..............................................................................................................................

..............................................................................................................................

..............................................................................................................................

..............................................................................................................................

..............................................................................................................................

..............................................................................................................................

..............................................................................................................................

..............................................................................................................................

..............................................................................................................................

..............................................................................................................................

..............................................................................................................................

..............................................................................................................................

..............................................................................................................................

# Month One

DAYS SINCE LAST PERIOD:_____

| EXERCISE |
| --- |
| |

| FOOD |
| --- |
| |

| OTHER SELF-CARE |
| --- |
| |

| | | DAY 1 | DAY 2 | DAY 3 | DAY 4 | DAY 5 |
|---|---|---|---|---|---|---|
| FLOW | LIGHT | | | | | |
| | MEDIUM | | | | | |
| | HEAVY | | | | | |
| COLOR | RED | | | | | |
| | PINK | | | | | |
| | RUSTY | | | | | |
| | OTHER | | | | | |

Use this chart to track your period patterns. We encourage you to write directly in the book! There are four more months starting on page 112, but if you'd like to track your period for longer, you can photocopy this page or copy it into a journal or notebook.

|  |  | DAY 1 | DAY 2 | DAY 3 | DAY 4 | DAY 5 |
|---|---|---|---|---|---|---|
| SYMPTOMS | CRAMPS | | | | | |
| | HEADACHE | | | | | |
| | TENDER BREASTS | | | | | |
| | BLOATING | | | | | |
| | DIARRHEA | | | | | |
| | ACNE | | | | | |
| | OTHER | | | | | |
| EMOTIONS | HAPPY | | | | | |
| | SAD | | | | | |
| | SENSITIVE | | | | | |
| | ANGRY | | | | | |
| | ANXIOUS | | | | | |
| | OTHER | | | | | |
| NOTES | | | | | | |

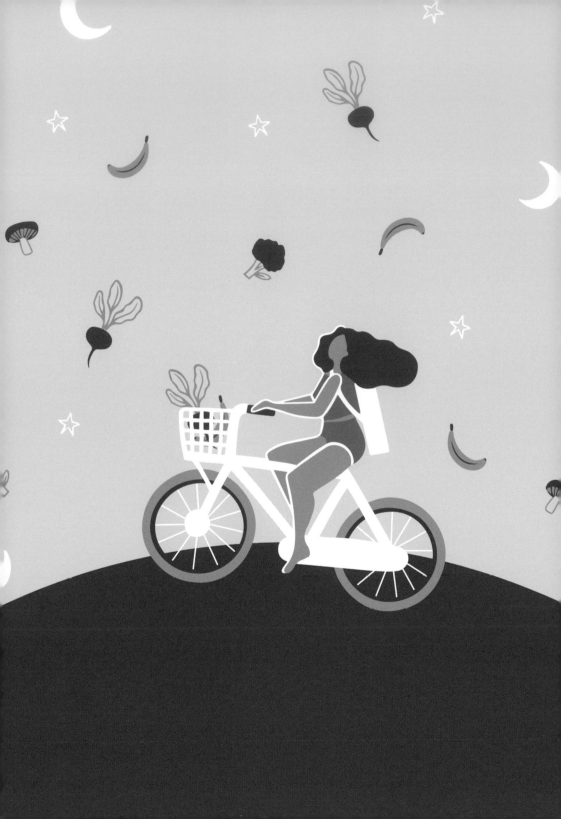

# Connect with Your Cycle

Nature is full of cycles—the cycle of the tides, the cycle of the seasons, the cycle of night and day. Your period is one of those natural cycles. But in the modern era, it's easy to feel disconnected from these natural ebbs and flows. In this chapter we'll look at how our personal cycles can be analogous to the cycle of the seasons, so that we can try to get back in touch with the rhythms of nature.

# Sync Your Cycle

Your hormone levels are constantly shifting throughout the different phases of your menstrual cycle. The phases are comparable to the four seasons in our environment: winter, spring, summer, and autumn.

Just as we need to adjust our routines to the outer seasons, we can also adjust to the inner seasons of our cycle. To balance the ebb and flow of hormones during these inner seasons, you can adjust your diet and lifestyle.

If you don't have a menstrual cycle due to contraception, menopause, hysterectomy, or any other reason, you can still sync your inner seasons by aligning with the lunar cycle. In that case your inner winter starts with the new moon, which focuses on releasing and shedding the old. And your inner summer starts with the full moon, which is all about manifestation and creation.

You are unique and so is your cycle, so you can always adjust these guidelines to make them work for you. But like everything else in nature, your body, your emotions, your needs, and your period are all in some way cyclical and analogous to other natural cycles. Honoring these internal seasons will help you know when to go easy on yourself and when to push a little harder.

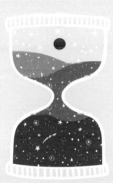

# The Four Seasons of the Cycle

Like the outer seasons, the inner seasons may sometimes be shorter or longer than average. If this is true for you, don't feel discouraged. The important thing is to become attuned to your own inner climate and your individual cycle.

## INNER WINTER (MENSTRUATION): FIRST QUARTER OF YOUR CYCLE

Your inner winter starts with the onset of menstruation and lasts until you stop menstruating. This season can often come with deep sadness but, being winter, it's also an opportunity to get cozy. Inner winter invites us to slow down, take a step back, maybe even burrow. This is your time to look inward, focusing on nourishment. This is a moment to give to yourself and not to others. Supportive rituals to do during your inner winter include journaling, taking baths, being in nature, and taking things slow so you can tap into your wisdom and creativity.

## INNER SPRING (PRE-OVULATION): SECOND QUARTER OF YOUR CYCLE

The time right before ovulation corresponds to the inner spring, which is all about fresh new energy starting to rise. It's the season of starting to move again, bringing more dynamic aspects into your daily life. This is the time when you want to get back into the world, when you may start to pick up projects, organize, and plan. As hormones begin to increase, you might notice that you are more productive and resilient. Spring stands for rebirth, starting anew, and productivity.

## INNER SUMMER (OVULATION): THIRD QUARTER OF YOUR CYCLE

Ovulation is closely connected to the season of summer, which is all about creation, manifestation, and procreation. It's a time of looking outward, of celebration and extroversion. This is the time to pick up social activities and to shine your light onto others. As radiance is connected to this season, so are power and strength. It is in your inner summer that you are most confident and you can ask for what you want in personal or work relationships. This season stands for playfulness, expression, relationship building, lovemaking, and creation.

## INNER AUTUMN (POST-OVULATION): FOURTH QUARTER OF YOUR CYCLE

After summer you might feel the urge to turn inward again. Autumn is a season of nesting; whether or not you actually ovulate, your body is preparing a space for an ovum to land. Since you're experiencing a natural inclination to turn inward, you might feel easily agitated when outside demands continue to build up. This is the season of starting to slow down and directing your energy toward drawing, poetry, or coming up with new ideas. You might feel moodier, as you crave some more space for yourself, and be more mentally creative.

# Eat According to Your Cycle

You probably already adjust your diet to the outer seasons; you may choose to eat seasonal produce, or favor stews in winter and salads in summer. Similarly, you can adjust your diet to the season of your inner cycle. Because you go through all four inner seasons about once a month, the inner and outer seasons will often be different. If it is winter outside while your cycle is in inner summer, look for a nice balance.

**Inner winter:** Warm and easily digestible food, more protein and fats. Focus on tastes like sweet, sour, and salty.

*Consider:* lentils, nuts, sesame seeds, leafy greens, eggs, walnuts, almond butter, honey, ghee,quinoa, beans, ginger, lemon, cinnamon, turmeric, cloves, black pepper.

**Inner spring:** Light and vibrant foods that kindle your inner sun.

*Consider:* ground flax seeds, organic tofu, pumpkin seeds, oats, colorful veggies, chili peppers, eggs, avocado, olive oil, bananas, onions, broccoli.

**Inner summer:** Foods that are cooling and high in water content—think salads, smoothies, juices, and fresh fruit.

*Consider:* leafy greens, almonds, cinnamon, sunflower and sesame seeds, whole grains, avocado, whole fruit, ginger tea, peppermint tea, water, coconut water, aloe vera juice.

**Inner autumn:** Roasted or baked root vegetables, foods high in fiber, greater calorie intake.

*Consider:* cauliflower, broccoli, brussels sprouts, garlic, hemp seeds, almonds, quinoa, berries, sunflower seeds, bell peppers, spinach.

# LIST YOUR FAVORITE FOODS
## FOR EACH INNER SEASON.

......................................................................................................

......................................................................................................

......................................................................................................

......................................................................................................

......................................................................................................

......................................................................................................

......................................................................................................

......................................................................................................

......................................................................................................

......................................................................................................

......................................................................................................

......................................................................................................

......................................................................................................

# Exercise with Your Cycle

Because you may have different amounts and types of energy during different inner seasons, it's important to take your cycle into account when choosing your workout routine.

**Inner winter:** Your hormone levels are at their lowest. Honor this by bringing a softer, gentler approach to your exercise routine. Think about meditation, walking, being out in nature, yin yoga, yoga nidra, and rest. For more inspiration, go to page 68, where we discuss yoga during menstruation.

**Inner spring:** Hormones and energy levels start to pick up! Focus on cardio-based workouts such as running, biking, dancing, and swimming.

**Inner summer:** Since your hormones are peaking, you can do more challenging workouts. Kickboxing, HIIT, power yoga, or bootcamps can be just what you need during your inner summer.

**Inner autumn:** Strength-based workouts are super supportive during your inner autumn. Think weightlifting, Pilates, and yoga.

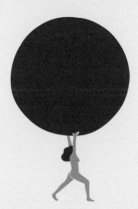

# LIST YOUR FAVORITE EXERCISES
## FOR EACH INNER SEASON.

# WHICH IS YOUR FAVORITE INNER SEASON, AND WHY?

........................................................................................

........................................................................................

........................................................................................

........................................................................................

........................................................................................

........................................................................................

........................................................................................

........................................................................................

........................................................................................

........................................................................................

........................................................................................

........................................................................................

........................................................................................

........................................................................................

# WHICH SEASON FEELS LEAST COMFORTABLE TO YOU? WHAT CAN YOU DO TO MAKE IT EASIER?

.................................................................................................

.................................................................................................

.................................................................................................

.................................................................................................

.................................................................................................

.................................................................................................

.................................................................................................

.................................................................................................

.................................................................................................

.................................................................................................

.................................................................................................

.................................................................................................

.................................................................................................

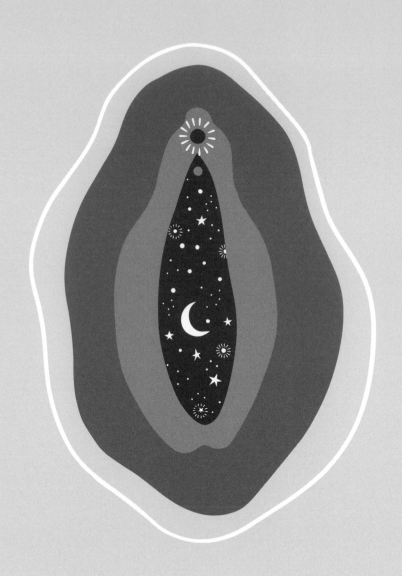

# Period
# Talk

Now it's time for us to talk about all the nitty-gritty details of your period! And not just talk—it's also time to look, feel, and observe. In this chapter, we'll get familiar with the specifics of menstruation and how they play out in your personal period. That means we're going to be talking about things some people see as unmentionable, like blood, mucus, and poop. But remember, there's no shame in your flow! All of this, even the poop, is a natural and normal part of life.

# Hormones in Check

If you don't feel sad, irritable, anxious, achy, tired, or generally bad around your period, count yourself lucky! Many people have emotional and physical effects from fluctuating hormones before menstruation (known as PMS), during menstruation, and at ovulation. How do you know if your hormones are playing havoc with you? Use this checklist to see how many signs of healthy hormone balance you have right now.

☐ Mental clarity

☐ Overall feeling of being content and joyful

☐ Steady energy level

☐ Emotional balance

☐ Typical sex drive for you

☐ Moist and lubricated vagina

☐ Sufficient sleep

☐ Active metabolism

☐ Stable weight

☐ Regular cycle if you menstruate

If you ticked more than eight of the boxes, you are a healthy, balanced hormonal hero and you can stop reading this book right now. (Just kidding—we'll discuss other things that will be relevant to you!) If you checked between five and eight, read on—you'll find many tips and tricks in this book to support your efforts to find greater balance. But even if you checked fewer than five, don't worry! You've come to the right place. We hope to give you the tools to understand your body, commune with your cycle, and achieve greater harmony—including hormone harmony. (If you need more help or guidance, though, please consult with your doctor.)

# Feeling Fiery

In Ayurveda, blood is said to contain a lot of the fire element. The qualities associated with the fire element are *hot*, *light*, *flowing*, and *sharp*.

Over the course of your cycle, blood builds up in the uterus as your uterine lining thickens, which means there's a buildup of the fire element within your body. Unless you make nutrition and lifestyle choices that counter this buildup, you could end up with an excess of fire at the end of your cycle, leading to:

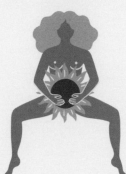

* IRRITABILITY

* DIARRHEA

* STINGING HEADACHE

* HOT FLASHES

* ACNE

What can you do to prevent excess fire?

**Lifestyle:** Chill out, relax, empty your agenda—you get the idea.

**Nutrition:** Refrain from consuming alcohol, fried foods, and foods that are very salty, sour, or pungent.

# HOW DO THE FIRE ELEMENT AND ITS CHARACTERISTICS MANIFEST IN YOUR LIFE?

# That Slimy Stuff

Vaginal discharge is normal! We should print this on a T-shirt.

All openings of the body have some kind of waste product. Think about earwax, or the gunk in your eyes when you wake up. For a vagina, those secretions include blood and vaginal discharge, also known as the slimy stuff you may see traces of in your underwear.

Vaginal discharge is made up of cervical mucus, vaginal secretions (including the ones that keep you lubricated during sex), and dead skin cells—it's part of your vagina's natural cleaning system! Most of the discharge is made up of cervical mucus, which has a role in fertility; that's why you'll probably see changes in the texture of your discharge over the course of your cycle.

**Nonfertile phase (period to ovulation):** Discharge during this phase may be dry, with barely any fluid, or it may be sticky, with a tacky texture, and may also be whitish and cloudy.

**Fertile phase (ovulation to period):** Discharge during this phase might be creamy and seem like a thicker whitish fluid, or it may have an egg-white texture and be a stretchy, slippery, and clear fluid.

The color and smell of your vaginal discharge can reveal a lot about your overall health! Normal vaginal discharge is whitish, not smelly, and has one of the textures discussed above. Signs of abnormal discharge include a strong or foul smell, itchy sensations, and pain. If you suffer from these, see a health professional.

# Period Poop

Finally, our favorite topic.

You might have noticed that just before, during, and just after your period, you experience a certain amount of gastrointestinal chaos. From a holistic point of view, this is connected to the buildup of blood, and therefore of fire, that we discussed on page 44. Diarrhea is one of the possible effects of too much fire in your system.

What can you do to avoid period poop?

* Reduce your stress levels. Stress is the number one way to increase the element of fire.
* Avoid foods that are very salty, sour, or pungent.
* Stay away from fried food.
* Make time for self-care.
* Spend time in nature, especially near water.

# Missing or Scanty Flow

There are other reasons besides pregnancy why your period might be very light or absent, chief among them stress.

In Ayurvedic practice, the wind element is responsible for the downward movement of menstrual blood. When there is a lot of activity in the mind—in other words, a lot of stress—the wind element will be disturbed, blowing turbulently around instead of in one steady stream. This leads to a diminished downward flow. Wind is also associated with the qualities of *drying*, *lightness* and *cooling*, qualities that in excess aren't good for internal tissues—we want those to be warm, robust, moist, and soft.

So what causes turmoil in your inner winds or an excess of wind element? Possible culprits include drastic weight change, physical and emotional stress, illness, and certain medications. (Remember that it's not unusual for hormonal contraception to make you skip a period—and you can always talk to your doctor about period changes.)

## HOW TO HARMONIZE

If you're experiencing an internal windstorm, nourishment and rest will be the keys to achieving harmony. Find a way to naturally anchor the inner winds so you can stop being buffeted around.

Internally, you can do this by adding more oils to your diet, such as ghee, olive oil, and avocado oil. You also want to bring in more mushy, warm, soft foods and earthy vegetables. Spice it up with cardamom, cinnamon, turmeric, cloves, and nutmeg.

Externally, you can anchor your inner winds with a warm sesame oil massage. Massage your torso from top to bottom, focusing on downward movement. You can also apply castor oil packs in the days leading up to menstruation. (See page 59 for instructions.)

# Heavy Periods

When the fire and water elements in your system are too great, your cycle may be very intense and come with heavy bleeding. You may experience tender, swollen breasts or have loose bowel movements and diarrhea.

## HOW TO HARMONIZE

Avoid competitive, challenging activities, which can overstimulate the fire element. If an activity makes your blood boil, even in a positive way—stay away from it during your period!

Choose cooling foods such as coconut oil, mint, chamomile, coriander, lavender, and leafy greens over rich, oily, spicy, and salty foods. You can use organic aloe vera juice to counterbalance the heating qualities of blood, since aloe vera is considered a cooling tonic. You only need to drink about an ounce, once in the morning and once at night.

Consult with your health practitioner to find other holistic herbs that can support you during a heavy flow.

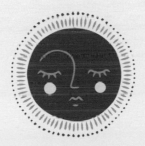

# Slow Cycle

If water and earth are the predominant elements in your constitution, then you may have a slow and stagnant cycle. When the elements of water and earth mix they become mud, which makes it harder for things to move. This often leads to water retention, swelling around the belly, bloating, and slow bowel movement. During the entire cycle, you may feel a deep craving to retreat and cocoon. Feel free to indulge these urges during the first days of your period! Eventually, though, you will want to reemerge and reactivate to prevent your body from staying in a lethargic state.

## HOW TO HARMONIZE

To counterbalance the natural sluggishness and lethargy of this combination of elements, you will need movement, activation, lightness, and warmth. So your mantra here is to spice things up!

Spice things up in the kitchen by adding more cinnamon, cardamom, tulsi, turmeric, ginger, black pepper, cayenne, and asafetida. Avoid dairy and moist, rich, sticky, heavy, oily, or overly sweet food.

Bring heat to the body through warm sesame oil self-massage (not too much oil, though—just a thin layer), hot baths, steams, and castor oil packs.

Spice things up internally with free movement, Ashtanga or power yoga practice, yogic breathing, brisk walks, cycling, running, hiking, and dry brushing (running a natural-fiber brush over the skin in circular motions, moving from the feet upward and always brushing toward the heart; this is thought to be an excellent way to stimulate tissues and activate the lymphatic system).

## WHICH OF THE AYURVEDIC ELEMENTS ON PAGE 9 DO YOU THINK IS PREDOMINANT FOR YOU? HOW DOES THAT AFFECT YOUR PERIOD?

51

# PMS Guide

Premenstrual syndrome, or PMS, has become a catch-all term for the various discomforts we may experience in the week or so before menstruation. These symptoms may be sporadic and minor, or they may return every month, keeping you from your daily activities. If your PMS symptoms are consistently disruptive, you may want to talk to your doctor about premenstrual dysphoric disorder, a more severe form of PMS.

We've listed some PMS symptoms here, along with nutrition and lifestyle advice to manage them. The list is far from complete. But it can direct you toward a holistic way of thinking about your PMS symptoms.

## PMS SYMPTOMS ASSOCIATED WITH A SCANTY FLOW

* LOWER BACK OR BELLY PAIN

* ANXIETY

* FEAR

* INSOMNIA

* BLOATING

**Do:** rest, relax, and try to find routine in your day-to-day life; eat warm, mushy foods, like soups and stews, with plenty of oil; try oil massages; drink plenty of water.

**Don't:** keep yourself too busy; have a chaotic lifestyle without routine, eat too many raw foods or dry foods like rice cakes and crackers, consume refrigerated fizzy drinks or too much caffeine.

# PMS SYMPTOMS ASSOCIATED WITH A HEAVY FLOW

* IRRITABILITY

* SENSITIVE BREASTS

* HOT FLASHES

* ACNE

* DIARRHEA

**Do:** take it easy; put a smile on your face; eat fresh fruits and vegetables, preferably green leafy vegetables; have some aloe vera juice.

**Don't:** get stressed or competitive, take things too seriously, eat spicy or fried foods, drink alcohol.

# PMS SYMPTOMS ASSOCIATED WITH A STAGNANT FLOW

* WATER RETENTION

* FEELING LETHARGIC

* DEPRESSION

**Do:** stay active, wake up early, eat light, use warming spices to ignite your inner fire.

**Don't:** oversleep, binge on sugary or salty processed foods, become a couch potato.

## WHAT PERIOD AND PMS SYMPTOMS
## GIVE YOU THE MOST TROUBLE?

## WHAT CAN YOU DO TO
## HARMONIZE YOUR PERIOD?

......................................................................................................

......................................................................................................

......................................................................................................

......................................................................................................

......................................................................................................

......................................................................................................

......................................................................................................

......................................................................................................

......................................................................................................

......................................................................................................

......................................................................................................

......................................................................................................

55

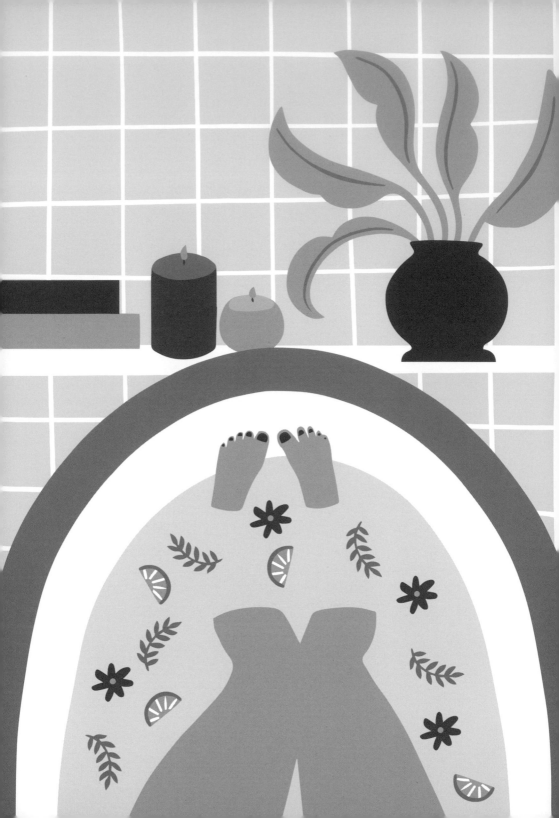

# Natural Self-Care

Especially during your period, when you may experience mental and physical discomfort, it's important to make time to care for, nurture, and love yourself. In this chapter we'll lay out some natural self-care activities developed in accordance with Ayurvedic principles. You can test them all out, or choose one that most speaks to you and incorporate it into your existing self-care routine.

# Castor Oil Pack

Castor oil, a vegetable oil made from castor beans, has been used as a natural remedy for literally thousands of years. It's been used to treat constipation, inflammation, and skin problems, to promote wound healing, and to help induce labor. And, most relevant for our purposes, it can help ease stagnant or scanty periods and promote better flow. If your period is irregular or insufficient, apply a castor oil pack three to four days before you are due to start menstruating, or three to four days before the new moon if you want to kick-start menstruation but don't currently have a cycle.

See page 60 for instructions on how to make a castor oil pack—but be warned, this can be a messy endeavor! Plan to do your castor oil pack at a time when you have time, space, and solitude to prepare carefully, relax for up to half an hour, and clean up thoroughly afterward.

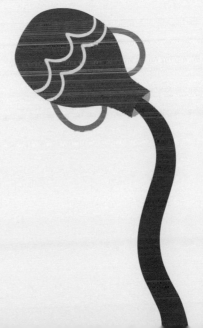

## YOU'LL NEED

* Cold-pressed castor oil (watch out, it's very sticky!)

* A piece of cotton big enough to cover your lower belly

* Old clothes or a towel to lie on (to prevent stains)

* A hot-water bottle

1   Massage some room-temperature (not cold) castor oil onto your abdomen.

2   Pour some castor oil on the cotton cloth.

3   Lie on an old towel and place the cloth on your abdomen, covering the area from your navel to your pubic bone.

4   Place the hot-water bottle over the cloth.

5   Lie down for twenty to thirty minutes. It's very nice to do this in your bed, with your legs against the wall.

The best time to apply a castor oil pack is in the evening, because it will probably make you sleepy. Note: never use castor oil during your period! Using this oil before your period stimulates your flow and reduces stagnation, but once the flow is happening you should relax and rely on your body's inner wisdom.

# Breast Massage

Because of the rise in hormones after ovulation, some people experience tender and swollen breasts before their period. It may help to massage your breasts with castor oil, which has anti-inflammatory properties and can help stimulate lymph circulation.

Since this oil is super sticky, you can apply it in the shower. Massage each breast for at least a minute.

As you massage your breasts one by one, you may also want to send some words or thoughts of positive affirmation and gratitude to your breasts and your body.

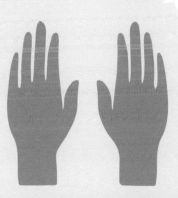

# Yoni Steam

A yoni steam is what it sounds like: allowing herbal steam to gently flow over your yoni. It's a beautiful restorative practice that balances the cycle and helps you reconnect to your uterus. A yoni steam is also used to ease cramps, aid fertility, and soothe the area after a miscarriage or birth. Depending on the purpose of the steam session, you may choose different herbs for your steam. For PMS, try a combination of mugwort, oregano, raspberry leaf, and red rose petals.

1   Boil 1 to 2 quarts of water in a saucepan.

2   Add your herbs to the boiling water and let sit for 10 minutes.

3   Now pour the mixture into a jar or bowl, and place the jar in your toilet.

4   Wait until the steam is not too hot to hold your hand over, then sit on the toilet. The water should not touch your buttocks.

5   Put on some music, wrap a blanket around your pelvic area, and sit for 10 to 20 minutes. Try to breathe into your vagina and uterus.

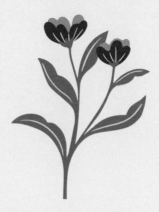

# Headache Release

If you've had acupuncture or acupressure therapy, you may be familiar with the idea that certain points on your skin are connected to energy pathways within the body, and that it's possible to influence physical and mental health by manipulating these points in some way. In Ayurveda, these are called marma points. Stimulating the marma points can help regulate the flow of prana throughout the body.

A few of these points are very useful in the treatment of menstrual discomfort. The marma points we personally use the most are the ones that help relieve headaches. The two points are located on either side of the head, at the temples. Feel for a fingertip-size depression that's roughly in line with the top of your ear. Massage these hollow spots with your index and middle finger for a few minutes to lessen any headache, including ones associated with your period. We like to use a bit of sandalwood oil for this.

Another Ayurvedic method of headache relief is a ritual gesture, or mudra, called the Great Head mudra. This is best performed while sitting comfortably, with a straight spine. Rest the backs of your hands on your thighs, so your palms are facing the ceiling. On each hand, press your thumb together with your middle and index finger. Tuck in your ring finger so it touches at the base of your thumb, but keep your pinky straight. Focus your breath and hold the mudra for at least five minutes.

# Good Flow
# Tummy Massage

If your cramps aren't too bad, try easing them with a tummy massage instead of immediately reaching for a painkiller. It's an opportunity to be fully present with an uncomfortable bodily sensation, sitting with it and observing it rather than trying to erase it. Our hands are instruments we often use to show affection and love for others. Can you also give yourself that same affection? This ritual for tummy massage will help soothe the discomfort in a mindful and self-loving way. This can also be used to bring in more downward movement to stimulate a lighter flow.

1    Rub your hands together to create some heat and energy.

2    Rest your hands on your belly, wherever you're experiencing the most discomfort.

3    Inhale, sending healing energy through your hands into your belly. Exhale to release discomfort and tension, and to relax. Repeat for five full inhales and exhales.

4    Start moving the right hand clockwise for about two minutes, massaging the abdominal wall, applying the pressure that feels right for you.

5    Now take four fingers of each hand and make little circles, massaging the abdomen with a bit more precision. Start far away from your navel and slowly spiral toward it. Again, you can adjust the pressure to your liking.

6    To seal the practice, rub your hands again to create some heat. Place them in the same spot where you started.

7    Take a few more deep breaths. Has anything shifted?

# Rest to Digest

In these busy modern times, it's easy to forget to take a rest—or even to feel bad about resting. But of all the health advice in this book, the most important is probably "get the rest you need." Nothing else you can do for your body or mind can take the place of adequate rest!

Societal pressure to constantly push ourselves, and to feel beholden to the demands of artificial systems (like work) instead of our natural rhythms, tends to alienate us from our bodies. Tuning in to your cycle can help reconnect you with your body's needs, including rest. Because your period is a time when your body cleanses and resets itself, it can be a reminder to take time to relax.

It's also especially important to rest during menstruation in order to support digestion—or, as we might say in Ayurveda, to help stoke your digestive fire. Ayurveda conceptualizes a fire within the body that helps with digestion and metabolism. During your period, you may find you have less digestive capacity. (Literally *and* figuratively—in holistic health, we say that it is not only food that needs to be digested, but also all the impressions you receive during the day through your senses.) On days that your digestive fire is reduced, treat it as you would a real fire that was getting low—give it easily consumed fuel, but don't smother it! Eat foods that are easy to digest, don't strain or push your body, and don't overload your sense organs in any way.

Let rest be your medicine!

# Honor Your Instincts

We have been teaching yoga classes, workshops, and retreats for quite a few years now, and what we've seen is that people frequently act against their bodies' natural instincts. Sometimes they're alienated from their physical needs because of the distractions and responsibilities of their hectic lifestyle. Other times, the unwritten rules of modern society encourage them to prioritize others' needs or the needs of impersonal systems over their own. Either way, people end up in conflict and confusion with their own bodies.

Instead, we encourage you to tune in to your instincts. Notice what makes you feel a strong internal sense of "yes" or "no," and honor that response— even when someone or something else may be pushing you to resist.

To give you some practical examples: Imagine you are on your period, and your body feels tired and needs rest. At 6 p.m., you are supposed to go to a bootcamp class with a friend. You don't want to cancel because of your period, because you've seen so many messages telling you that periods aren't important or that resting is a sign of weakness. Your body is clearly saying "no" to strenuous exercise, but societal cues tell you to tough it out.

Or: You're not on your period yet, but you will probably start tomorrow. You're starting to feel a little crampy and fatigued. Your instincts are telling you to stay home with tea and Netflix. But hey, it's Friday night, and your friends are going out drinking. You'd feel like a party pooper if you bailed. Your body is saying "yes" when you think about taking it easy, but social pressure makes you unwilling to break plans.

The whole idea of cycles—menstrual cycles, the cycle of seasons, the cycle of a day, and the other cycles in our lives—is that they're *cyclical*. Sometimes you're on an upward swing, and you feel inspired, enthusiastic, and vibrant. Sometimes the energy is downward, and you feel slower and more reserved. You can't be at peak energy all the time— and if you try, eventually you'll find that it's unbalanced and unhealthy.

# WHAT CAN YOU DO TO HONOR
# YOUR INNER "YES" AND "NO"?

# Yoga During Your Cycle

Namaste! Yoga is close to our hearts, because yoga and Ayurveda are closely connected—they're both systems of Vedic knowledge, Indian philosophy with ancient roots. Ayurveda focuses on healing, while yoga is a spiritual practice. The physical postures you might do in yoga class are only a small part of yoga! But that's the part we'll be focusing on here.

So, is it a good idea to do yoga during your period? The answer is: yes and no. (This is the answer to a lot of questions, when you look at them from a holistic point of view.) Some types of yoga and some postures are helpful when you're menstruating, and others are better saved for a different point in your cycle.

As we've said throughout this book, your period is a time to take it slow. We encourage you to avoid anything that puts too much strain on your body. However, gentle, mindful movement can help to relieve cramping and remove blockages, both physically and energetically. (What *gentle* means will be a little different for everyone, so start slow and ramp up incrementally to discover your level of comfort.)

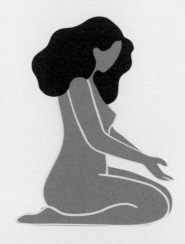

## POSTURES TO AVOID

* Any postures where your legs are up and the hips are higher than the heart. For instance, downward dog is just fine—the hips are higher than the heart, while the legs are downward—but avoid a headstand or shoulder stand.

* Any movements that are fast and erratic.

## POSTURES TO TRY

* Butterfly, both seated and lying down
* Child's pose
* Gentle twists
* Forward folds
* Deep breathing
* Cat/cow

# Gone with the Wind

Apana vayu is an Ayurvedic concept meaning downward-moving wind. And this energetic downward force is one of the most important factors in your physical and mental well-being.

Downward-moving wind helps with:

* PEEING AND POOPING

* DELIVERING BABIES

* FEELING GROUNDED

* MENSTRUATING

In order to keep apana vayu moving smoothly in the right direction, make sure you're not suppressing your natural urges. (Yes, we mean you should be letting those farts fly.)

During menstruation, it's especially important that the downward wind is allowed to flow without any blockages. One way to achieve this, from a holistic point of view, is to make sure your hips are not higher than your heart, which would hamper the natural downward flow. Keep this in mind when choosing exercises and yoga poses during your period—for instance, handstands, glute bridges, and Pilates bicycles all invert the downward movement. It's okay to temporarily have your hips higher than your heart, but avoid holding these postures for a longer time.

## WHICH SELF-CARE PRACTICE SPEAKS
## TO YOU MOST, AND WHY?

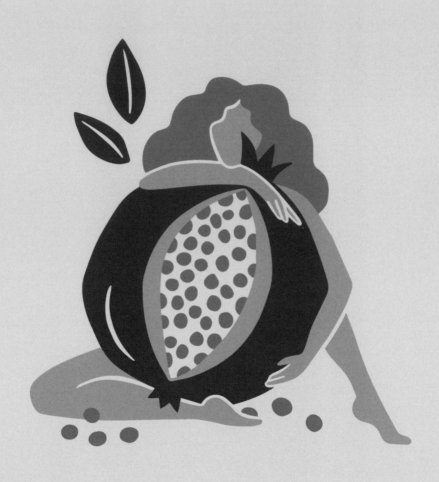

# Boost Your Power

You are what you eat—so if you don't eat enough, how can you be enough? When we deplete or undernourish our bodies, we can expect to see consequences to our health and energy levels. But when we take in nourishing foods, we can build strength and resilience—including healthy menstruation.

# Iron (Wo)Man

Heavy bleeding during your period can lead to iron deficiency. Symptoms of iron deficiency (also called anemia) include fatigue, weakness, poor concentration, shortness of breath, lightheadedness, and pallor.

If you think you may be clinically iron deficient, you may want to talk to a doctor about supplements. But if you need a boost to your iron levels just during menstruation, choosing iron-rich foods may help you feel stronger and more energetic. Foods with high iron content include:

* LIVER

* SHELLFISH

* CARROTS

* RAISINS

* BEETS

* SPINACH

* POMEGRANATES

* FIGS

* PUMPKIN SEEDS

* QUINOA

* DATES

# Seed Cycling

Eating different seeds during the menstrual cycle can help improve PMS symptoms and irregular hormone levels. All you need are two glass jars, one for seeds to eat during the first half of your cycle and one for the second half. Fill the jars as follows:

**New moon mix (menstruation to ovulation):** Linseed and pumpkin seeds

**Full moon mix (ovulation to menstruation):** Sesame and sunflower seeds

Use two tablespoons of the appropriate seed mix daily. You can add them to your yogurt, smoothie, or salad, or sprinkle on top of anything you're eating.

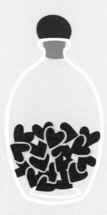

# Your Herbal Allies

Don't underestimate the power of herbs! The word might make you think of humble plants you use in cooking—but the right herbal supplements, with the right application and dosage, are also potent plant medicine. In fact, we recommend consulting with a natural health physician before using the menstruation-supporting herbs below. (You'll likely find these at a specialized store for herbal remedies, not at your grocery store with the dried dill!)

* Ashoka: Helps regulate the menstrual cycle. Also very useful for reducing period cramps.

* Shatavari: The name of this asparagus relative translates as "she who has one hundred husbands." It rejuvenates the reproductive organs.

* Maca: An adaptogenic herb that helps to regulate hormones. Also works as a libido booster.

* Musta: Supports a healthy and regular cycle and promotes digestion.

# Tend Your Digestive Fire

When you are menstruating, your digestive fire is low. During your period, you want to eat simple, easily digestible meals. Don't smother the fire with too much fuel—eat only when you're hungry and when the previous meal is fully digested. This can be a bit challenging if you're having hormone-induced cravings, but as you adjust your routine to your inner seasons and get more in tune with your inner rhythms, you'll find that cravings decrease.

For the first couple of days of your period, go for warm, mushy stews with your favorite veggies, rice, and some nice nourishing homemade banana bread. This truly will do wonders for your body, mind, and soul.

A few points to consider when eating during your period:

* Leave at least three hours between meals, to make sure that your previous meal is fully digested.

* Check in with your body—are you hungry, or are you bored or in need of a break?

* Only eat while sitting down.

* Eat in a calm environment—no screens, no distractions.

* Once you are satisfied, stop, even if there is still food on your plate.

* Chew thoroughly.

* Breathe.

## HAVE YOU USED FOOD AS MEDICINE BEFORE?
## HOW DID IT WORK FOR YOU?

...................................................................................................

...................................................................................................

...................................................................................................

...................................................................................................

...................................................................................................

...................................................................................................

...................................................................................................

...................................................................................................

...................................................................................................

...................................................................................................

...................................................................................................

...................................................................................................

...................................................................................................

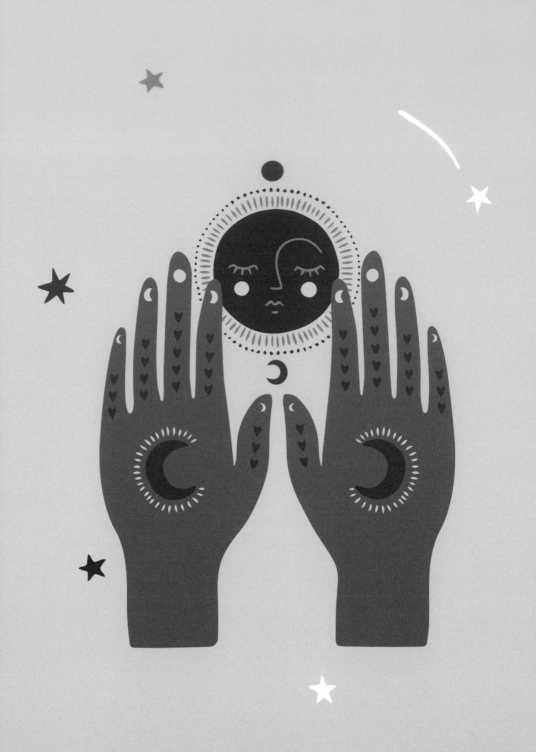

# Moon Rituals

**R**itual is a powerful tool for self-care—it allows you to set intentions, be fully present in the moment, and carve out time and space that's devoted to your own well-being. We've selected some Ayurvedic and Ayurveda-inspired ritual practices and meditations for period wellness, but we invite you to adapt and build on them in whatever way helps you in forging a closer connection to yourself and your body.

# Yoni Mudra

A mudra is a symbolic hand gesture. It aims to direct your energy and awareness within your body, enhancing the flow of prana. You can use mudras during meditation, during a yoga practice, or just during your day for a moment of centering and calm.

The yoni mudra targets the pelvis and uterus. It can help you deepen your connection with deep earth energies. It may also help to reduce stress and anxiety and balance hormones.

1   Bring your palms together in front of your body with the fingers pointing down.

2   Curl the ring, middle, and pinkie fingers inward, so that the backs of the fingers are touching. The thumbs and index fingers remain in place.

3   The index fingers should be pointing toward the pelvis region, and the thumbs pointing up toward the navel. The index fingers and thumb should form a diamond shape.

Once you've mastered yoni mudra, you can use it as part of a meditation (see the next page), or just rest your hands on your belly in this position and breathe for three to five minutes.

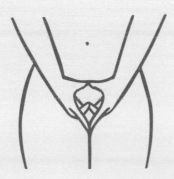

# Womb Meditation

This short meditation can be practiced at any time, but we recommend doing it in the morning to set the tone of your day.

1   Lie down on your back, with a pillow or blanket supporting your knees if you have lower back problems (or just feel more comfortable this way).

2   Place your hands in yoni mudra (see previous page).

3   Close your eyes and focus your awareness on your belly, as you place the yoni mudra onto your lower belly.

4   Consciously breathe into the mudra.

5   Once you feel connected and present, start to imagine you are breathing golden light into the womb space, allowing that area to fill up.

6   Then envision exhaling the light outward, radiating it into the universe.

7   Continue to envision inhaling and exhaling golden light for a couple of minutes. Observe how you feel.

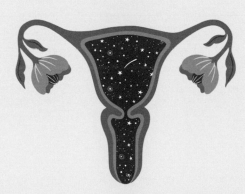

# Red Tent

Historically, some cultures have mandated that menstruating women must isolate in purpose-built lodges, tents, or menstruation huts. For some, this has overtones of exile or treating menstruation as taboo, but it was also an opportunity to withdraw from community responsibilities and devote time to introspection or spiritual practice.

In our modern world, it can be more difficult to retreat in this way. But you can emulate the positive parts of period isolation by consciously taking time for yourself while menstruating. If you cannot take time off from work, make sure not to pack your free time with social gatherings. On the contrary, mark out some me time to focus on how you can care for and nourish yourself. This is easier to plan in advance if you have a regular cycle, but even if your period is not predictable, give yourself permission to take time during those days to disengage.

# Beem Mantra

A mantra is a sound vibration that helps to direct thoughts and feelings. Bija mantras are simple, one-syllable mantras that are each attuned to a specific concept, element, deity, or part of the body. They're also called seed mantras because they are simple sounds that can be developed into something more complex. The bija mantra *beem* helps bring vibration, energy, and nourishment to the yoni and womb.

This mantra is very helpful to work with when you have an irregular cycle, you are trying to conceive, your cycle is too long, or you don't have a cycle and you want to recover it.

1  Sit on your heels, with a straight spine.

2  On each hand, touch your thumb with your middle and ring finger (this posture is called tattva mudra).

3  Set your timer for three to five minutes.

4  Place both of your hands over your ovaries.

5  Chant the mantra *beem* until the timer goes off.

6  Sit for a moment to observe and allow the magic to unfold.

# Saying Farewell to the Unfertilized Egg

If you are trying to get pregnant, your period may feel like a somber occasion. You may internalize messages that make you feel like you failed to conceive, even though it's notoriously a process with a great deal of luck involved! If you're feeling this way, it may be valuable to take some time to reflect on and honor the work your body does to make conception and childbirth possible. And if you're not trying to get pregnant, it's still worth taking some time during your cycle to appreciate all the work your body does for you..

Regardless of your personal choices about childbirth or parenthood, you have to appreciate how elegantly the human body provides for the perpetuation of the species. Even before you were born, your body contained all the egg cells you would ever have! Like clockwork (or slightly less like clockwork if your period isn't regular), your body sends out one egg a month for potential fertilization. When not pregnant, it keeps the womb clean by menstruating every month and then diligently rebuilds the uterine lining for the next attempt. And it does this without you having to do anything! It's easy to see menstruation as just an inconvenience, but it's also an amazing testament to the power and precision of the body.

Say this mantra silently or aloud to foster a deep connection to your reproductive organs, and to process whatever feelings you may be having about the passing of an unfertilized egg.

"Thank you, body, for tending to my womb, the place where life starts. Farewell to the egg that I have been carrying all my life, which now merges again with the earth."

# Journaling with Your Menstrual Cycle

Journaling is a beautiful way of organizing thoughts. It is an invitation to show up for yourself and to spend time introspecting and processing the events of your day. Keeping a journal over a longer period of time will give you ownership over your experiences. It is a way of reaching within yourself for answers, trusting that you hold all the needed wisdom within. To get you started we offer you some reflective questions and prompts for each stage in your cycle.

## DURING PERIOD

* Where am I at right now?

* What can I let go of?

* What new seeds can be planted?

* How can I nourish myself and bring in more compassion and grace?

* What does my inner wisdom want me to know?

## PERIOD TO OVULATION

* What do I want to bring into action this cycle?

* What new projects or opportunities do I feel attracted to?

* How can I show up this week and honor my priorities?

* Create some positive affirmations for new undertakings.

* Imagine yourself as a child. What does that child want to show you?

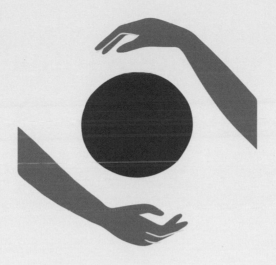

# OVULATION

* What can I celebrate right now?

* What am I grateful for?

* What is my deepest desire?

* What do I allow myself to receive right now?

* How can I slow down to listen to the wisdom inside me?

# OVULATION TO PERIOD

* What can I release?

* What limiting beliefs and fears are holding me back?

* What is draining my energy?

* How can I surrender?

* What boundaries are arising?

# New Moon Ritual

The new moon is the time of month when the moon presents its dark side to the earth, before it begins to wax toward full again. Your period is analogous to the new moon because it's a time of turning inward, evaluating what matters, releasing what doesn't serve you, and clearing space for new energy. A new moon ritual honors this time by directing your awareness inward, connecting you to what you need right now, and giving you permission to relinquish what you don't. You can see the new moon, or your period, as an opportunity to consciously release old patterns and create space to manifest new things.

Below you will find a simple ritual that can last anywhere from five to thirty minutes, depending on what you feel you need.

You will need: two pieces of paper, a pen, a smudge stick or other way to cleanse your space, a meditation pillow, a blanket, at least one candle, and matches or a lighter.

1   Prepare the space by gathering everything you need. Use the pillow and blanket to help yourself sit comfortably.

2   Dim the lights and light the candle or candles.

3   Smudge or otherwise cleanse the space.

4   Take a moment to center yourself with a womb meditation. You can use the one on page 84.

5   Once you feel centered and tuned in to your body, complete the following prompts, writing each down on a piece of paper:

   *   I release myself from . . .
   *   I will invite . . .

6   Fold the papers and sit in contemplation for another moment to connect to your message.

**7** Continue to meditate for as long as you wish, and conclude the ritual however feels right to you. The ritual can be considered over when you decide to end your meditation, or you can mark the end by burning the paper in the flame of the candle. (If you are going to burn paper, please do so outside in a safe area.)

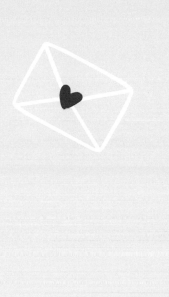

# Full Moon Ritual

The full moon is analogous to ovulation: a time of abundance and fullness. In the same way that the moon acts on the tides, the full moon amplifies what is alive in your heart, body, spirit, and mind. Positive and negative emotions alike are intensified, so you may want to channel this strong energy into a ritual.

This is a time to celebrate with others. So if you'd like to do this moon ritual with friends, go ahead; this is a wonderful way to raise collective consciousness.

You will need: speakers, your favorite dance playlist, a smudge stick or other way to cleanse your space, matches or a lighter, candles, paper and something to write with, and a glass bottle with filtered water.

1   Place the glass bottle of filtered water under the light of the full moon. Let this absorb the moon's energy for at least thirty minutes. In the meantime you can prepare the room for the ritual.

2   Prepare your space. Gather the items you need, dim the lights, and light the candles.

3   Smudge or otherwise cleanse the room.

4   Center yourself with a short meditation—you can use the womb meditation on page 84.

5   Put on your favorite playlist and start moving. Start by moving your spine, then let the movements travel out to your limbs and get bigger. Don't think about this; let the movement come from within.

6   When you're done moving, come to a slow stop. Take the time to feel and write down any thoughts and feelings that come up.

7   Drink the moon-infused water.

# USE THIS SPACE TO COME UP WITH YOUR OWN RITUAL HONORING AN ASPECT OF YOUR PERIOD.

# Red Fertilizer

Your body builds up your uterine lining in order to nourish life. If you're not using it that way, what about giving your plants a monthly mineral boost? Diluted period blood can be used to fertilize your plants—we recommend about one part blood to about eight to ten parts water.

We know a lot of people have a gross-out reaction to the concept of watering your plants with menstrual blood. Many of us are squeamish about anything that comes out of the human body, and that's largely for good reason—a lot of bodily secretions are waste products that could even cause disease. But some of that attitude also comes from the cultural idea that period blood is unclean, and that's simply not true! If you want to forge a deeper connection to your cycle and the natural world around you, and the idea of using period blood to nourish your plants appeals to you, you can do it without fear. Period blood is as nontoxic as any other blood. And you know what, it works really well as plant food!

# Facial Mask

If you came around on the idea of period plant food, here's a bigger challenge: a menstrual blood face mask. Wait, come back!

We get it—menstruation is still surrounded by a lot of shame, disgust, embarrassment, and secrecy. But that taboo is supported at least partly (if not completely!) by misogyny. Many patriarchal cultures think, openly or covertly, that vaginas and uteruses are, by their association with women, fundamentally suspicious and gross. That's why some feminist and women's empowerment movements encourage people to embrace and make use of their own menstrual blood, counteracting this cultural aversion.

One of those empowerment practices involves using your menstrual blood as a face mask. Period blood has anti-inflammatory benefits and is rich in stem cells and nutrients such as zinc, copper, and magnesium. (Although really, the purpose of the period blood mask is less about skin care and more about celebrating your cycle and refusing to submit to shame.)

Anointing yourself with menstrual blood is an invitation to connect to deep inner wisdom. Not everyone is going to be comfortable with this practice, but if it appeals, you may find that it's a surprisingly powerful experience. (Make sure you don't have any sexually transmitted infections first—some of these can be carried by period blood and you don't want to introduce them to the delicate membranes of the face.)

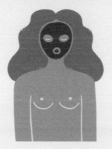

# Blood Drawing

What does it mean for something to be artistic, aesthetic, beautiful, or poetic? It's impossible to answer these questions objectively; that's what we mean by the expression "beauty is in the eye of the beholder." Every single one of us is an artist, and every single one of us has their own preferences about colors, forms, shapes, and other aspects of beauty.

Making art with menstrual blood is another way that people around the world are resisting stigma and shame and rediscovering menstruation as a source of power. It is a way of expressing the sacredness of blood, allowing the beauty of the cycle to come through, and shedding the idea of having to hide or be ashamed about menstruation. Especially when you are trying to conceive, menstrual art can be a very powerful ritual to embrace the cycle of nature. If you feel drawn to this practice, then try it out for yourself. Collect the blood in a menstrual cup or other receptacle and paint your emotions, your connection with the cycles of nature, or whatever you want to express right now.

## WHICH OF THE RITUALS IN THIS CHAPTER ARE YOU MOST DRAWN TO? WHICH RITUAL ARE YOU RESISTANT TO, AND WHY?

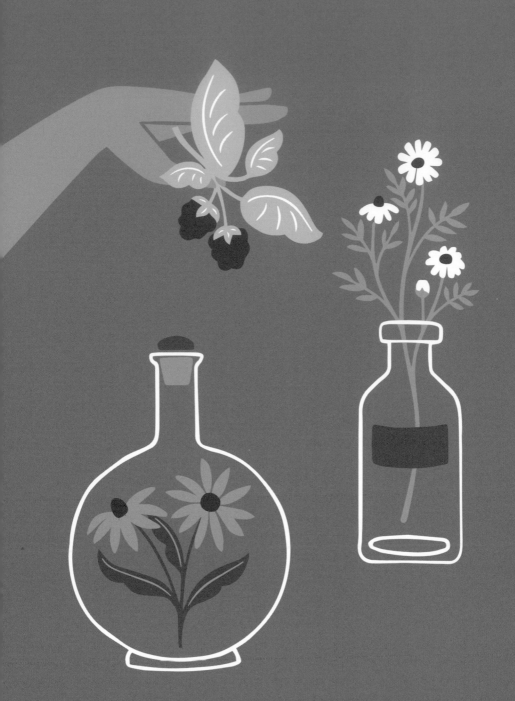

# Home
# Apothecary

**M**ost of us cook and eat for taste—we want something to taste good, and we may prioritize that over what something can do for our bodies. But if you open your kitchen cabinet right now, you will probably find plenty of items that can also be used as a medicine.

# Nourish Your Womb

Holistic medicine, and especially Ayurveda, looks at diet in a completely different way from Western medicine. We're not interested in counting calories or macronutrients, but in qualities of food and its action within the body. In Ayurveda, different foods have natural affinities with different parts of the body, and we can choose to eat foods corresponding with the parts of the body that need the most support.

The Ayurvedic view of food, flavor, and nutrition is complex, and you don't have to understand it all in order to eat well for your cycle! Suffice it to say that what you eat can have an effect on your menstruation, and choosing foods that support the uterus and its functioning can help you have a better period. The following foods have a natural affinity with the reproductive organs:

* MILK

* GHEE

* DATES

* ALMONDS

* SAFFRON

* HONEY

* SESAME SEEDS

* BASMATI RICE

* RAISINS

* ASPARAGUS

* OYSTERS

# Chocolate News

Having massive chocolate cravings on your period feels like a hackneyed joke, but it's a stereotype for a reason! Chocolate has many nutritional health benefits, and dark chocolate in particular is rich in magnesium, which can help relieve cramps by relaxing your muscles. The great news is, you don't need to suppress your desires for chocolate on your period. If you make good choices about quality and quantity, chocolate can bring you both physical and mental relief.

From a holistic perspective, there's no need to avoid sweets—the key is to prioritize quality. Low-quality sweets often have additives to enhance flavor, which can be more difficult to digest. This kind of sweet brings both dullness and chaos to the mind. High-quality sweets are natural and minimally processed. In moderation, high-quality sweets can bring clarity and openness.

Avoid chocolate bars made from primarily refined sugars and cacao butter—these won't get you the physical *or* mental benefits, and they may make you feel worse. Choose dark chocolate with a natural sweetener, like date sugar or coconut sugar. Or even better, go for something made in your own kitchen, such as the recipes in this chapter.

# Herbal Tonics

Medicines are not known for their great taste—but when you use food and herbs as your medicine, you don't need a spoonful of sugar to help it go down. These recipes help treat cramps and support menstruation *while* tasting great.

## HAPPY WOMB SHAKE

This warm, creamy shake supports uterine functioning (and tastes great).

### INGREDIENTS

* 8 ounces almond milk

* 1 Medjool date, pitted

* ⅛ teaspoon each of ground nutmeg, cardamom, and cinnamon

* A pinch of saffron

* ½ teaspoon ghee

Place the almond milk, date, and spices in a blender. Mix well. Transfer to a pan over medium-low heat and warm the mixture a little bit. Melt in the ghee. Enjoy!

# GENTLE PERIOD TEA

Drink this tea to help reduce or prevent menstrual cramps and excess bleeding. You should be able to find dried leaves and flowers at a tea shop, a spice shop, or an organic food store.

## INGREDIENTS

* Rose petals

* Raspberry leaves

* Red clover

* Hibiscus flowers

Fill a tea ball or loose tea bag with ½ teaspoon of each herb per cup of water, and steep in hot water for 2 to 3 minutes. During most of the month you can drink 1 cup of this light tea daily. During menstruation, use 1 teaspoon of the herbs and drink 1 quart of strong tea per day.

Important note: this tea should not be consumed during pregnancy. If you are trying to become pregnant, we also recommend not drinking this tea after ovulation.

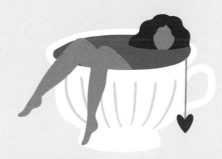

# Easy Tea Recipes

It's best to take a break from coffee during your period—which makes this time a wonderful opportunity to enter the miraculous world of tea. A cup of tea can give you an opportunity for a moment of rest and self-care, while also doubling as an herbal remedy. To make an herbal tea, use one to two tablespoons of herb per quart of hot water, and let it steep for two to three minutes for most herbs, or ten minutes for ginger.

**Rose:** Rose tea can offer some relief when you are suffering from period cramps. Start sipping it throughout the day beginning a week before your period is due.

**Ginger:** Very strong ginger tea can give instant relief from menstrual cramps.

**Nettle:** This pesky stinging plant has quite a few medicinal benefits. Nettle purifies the blood and eases heavy menstruation.

**Motherwort:** This antispasmodic herb can be used for painful cramps. It can also encourage a sluggish period, as its compounds help to stimulate blood flow and makes the uterine muscles contract.

**Chamomile:** This simple herb is also super powerful! It's known for its relaxing qualities, making it an essential tool for PMS anxiety. But it's also an antispasmodic, meaning it can help relieve muscle spasms like menstrual cramps.

**Cinnamon:** Cinnamon is loaded with antioxidants that can help lower inflammation. It has a high amount of manganese, which is helpful for alleviating PMS symptoms. And it can help with stomach pain, bloating, and indigestion, as long as you don't take too much.

**Raspberry leaf:** Tea made from raspberry leaf is a classic herbal remedy for periods and pregnancy. It can help strengthen the uterine muscles, ease period pains, and balance heavy bleeding.

# Moon Milk

Make this nourishing plant-based drink infused with adaptogens and spices when you want a reminder to slow down and take it easy. You can drink it daily before bedtime, or use it more ceremonially on period days.

## INGREDIENTS

* 8 ounces almond milk

* 1 tablespoon cacao powder

* ½ teaspoon ashwaganda powder (you can get this in a health food store)

* 4–5 rose petals

* 2–3 cardamom pods or ⅛ teaspoon ground cardamom

* ⅛ teaspoon pink salt

* ½ to 1 teaspoon raw honey (depending on your sweet tooth)

1  Heat milk to a simmer in a saucepan over medium heat.

2  Add cacao, ashwaganda, rose petals, cardamom, and salt. Whisk well while simmering. If the liquid seems like it's about to boil, lower the heat.

3    Once the milk is heated through, turn off heat, cover, and let sit for 3 minutes.

4    Pour into your favorite mug.

5    Let it cool down a little and then add honey. (Honey should never be added to beverages that are warmer than 70 degrees; at high heat it can lose some of its healthful properties and according to Ayurveda would be considered toxic.)

Increase the relaxing power of this concoction by drinking with intention, concentrating on the feeling of receiving nectar for your soul and your womb.

# Tropical Fruits

Mangoes, pineapples, papayas, avocados, and guavas aren't just among the tastiest fruits. Their sweet taste is also nourishing for your reproductive system!

Tropical fruits are packed with antioxidants, vitamin C, and vitamin B6, which are all vital to a healthy menstrual cycle. They are often high in fiber to aid digestion.

You don't need to eat these fruits daily or year-round; if you don't live in an area where they naturally grow, consuming tropical fruits can be expensive and environmentally unfriendly. But when they're available, try adding them to your period diet for their positive effects. Many of these fruits are also low on the list of pesticide contamination, so you can save money by buying conventional produce rather than organic.

## WHAT IS YOUR MAIN TAKEAWAY FROM THIS BOOK?

# WHAT NEW PRACTICES WOULD YOU LIKE TO INCORPORATE INTO YOUR LIFE?

# Follow Your Flow

Recording the details of your cycle and your physical and emotional symptoms can give you a better understanding of your period. It can also help you track how lifestyle factors like food, exercise, and self-care contribute to how you feel. As you implement the techniques from this book, you can use these charts and journal pages to observe how your cycle changes from month to month. Fill out the grids to see the details of your flow and accompanying symptoms at a glance, and use the blank pages to reflect on what's helping, what's still a challenge, and what you want to try next.

# Month Two

DAYS SINCE LAST PERIOD:_____

| EXERCISE |
|---|
| |

| FOOD |
|---|
| |

| OTHER SELF-CARE |
|---|
| |

| | | DAY 1 | DAY 2 | DAY 3 | DAY 4 | DAY 5 |
|---|---|---|---|---|---|---|
| **FLOW** | LIGHT | | | | | |
| | MEDIUM | | | | | |
| | HEAVY | | | | | |
| **COLOR** | RED | | | | | |
| | PINK | | | | | |
| | RUSTY | | | | | |
| | OTHER | | | | | |

Use this chart to track your period patterns. We encourage you to write directly in the book, but if you'd like to track your period for longer, we suggest you photocopy this page or copy it into a journal or notebook.

| | | DAY 1 | DAY 2 | DAY 3 | DAY 4 | DAY 5 |
|---|---|---|---|---|---|---|
| SYMPTOMS | CRAMPS | | | | | |
| | HEADACHE | | | | | |
| | TENDER BREASTS | | | | | |
| | BLOATING | | | | | |
| | DIARRHEA | | | | | |
| | ACNE | | | | | |
| | OTHER | | | | | |
| EMOTIONS | HAPPY | | | | | |
| | SAD | | | | | |
| | SENSITIVE | | | | | |
| | ANGRY | | | | | |
| | ANXIOUS | | | | | |
| | OTHER | | | | | |
| NOTES | | | | | | |

# Reflections on Month Two:

## WHAT WAS CHALLENGING?
## WHAT IMPROVED?
## WHAT CHANGES DO I WANT TO TRY?

# Month Three

DAYS SINCE LAST PERIOD:_____

| EXERCISE |
| --- |
| |

| FOOD |
| --- |
| |

| OTHER SELF-CARE |
| --- |
| |

| | | DAY 1 | DAY 2 | DAY 3 | DAY 4 | DAY 5 |
| --- | --- | --- | --- | --- | --- | --- |
| **FLOW** | LIGHT | | | | | |
| | MEDIUM | | | | | |
| | HEAVY | | | | | |
| **COLOR** | RED | | | | | |
| | PINK | | | | | |
| | RUSTY | | | | | |
| | OTHER | | | | | |

Use this chart to track your period patterns. We encourage you to write directly in the book, but if you'd like to track your period for longer, we suggest you photocopy this page or copy it into a journal or notebook.

|  |  | DAY 1 | DAY 2 | DAY 3 | DAY 4 | DAY 5 |
|---|---|---|---|---|---|---|
| SYMPTOMS | CRAMPS |  |  |  |  |  |
|  | HEADACHE |  |  |  |  |  |
|  | TENDER BREASTS |  |  |  |  |  |
|  | BLOATING |  |  |  |  |  |
|  | DIARRHEA |  |  |  |  |  |
|  | ACNE |  |  |  |  |  |
|  | OTHER |  |  |  |  |  |
| EMOTIONS | HAPPY |  |  |  |  |  |
|  | SAD |  |  |  |  |  |
|  | SENSITIVE |  |  |  |  |  |
|  | ANGRY |  |  |  |  |  |
|  | ANXIOUS |  |  |  |  |  |
|  | OTHER |  |  |  |  |  |
| NOTES | | | | | | |

# Reflections on Month Three:

## WHAT WAS CHALLENGING?
## WHAT IMPROVED?
## WHAT CHANGES DO I WANT TO TRY?

# Month Four

DAYS SINCE LAST PERIOD:_____

| EXERCISE |
| --- |
| |

| FOOD |
| --- |
| |

| OTHER SELF-CARE |
| --- |
| |

| | | DAY 1 | DAY 2 | DAY 3 | DAY 4 | DAY 5 |
| --- | --- | --- | --- | --- | --- | --- |
| FLOW | LIGHT | | | | | |
| | MEDIUM | | | | | |
| | HEAVY | | | | | |
| COLOR | RED | | | | | |
| | PINK | | | | | |
| | RUSTY | | | | | |
| | OTHER | | | | | |

Use this chart to track your period patterns. We encourage you to write directly in the book, but if you'd like to track your period for longer, we suggest you photocopy this page or copy it into a journal or notebook.

| | | DAY 1 | DAY 2 | DAY 3 | DAY 4 | DAY 5 |
|---|---|---|---|---|---|---|
| SYMPTOMS | CRAMPS | | | | | |
| | HEADACHE | | | | | |
| | TENDER BREASTS | | | | | |
| | BLOATING | | | | | |
| | DIARRHEA | | | | | |
| | ACNE | | | | | |
| | OTHER | | | | | |
| EMOTIONS | HAPPY | | | | | |
| | SAD | | | | | |
| | SENSITIVE | | | | | |
| | ANGRY | | | | | |
| | ANXIOUS | | | | | |
| | OTHER | | | | | |
| NOTES | | | | | | |

# Reflections on Month Four:

## WHAT WAS CHALLENGING?
## WHAT IMPROVED?
## WHAT CHANGES DO I WANT TO TRY?

# Month Five

DAYS SINCE LAST PERIOD:_____

| EXERCISE |
| --- |
| |

| FOOD |
| --- |
| |

| OTHER SELF-CARE |
| --- |
| |

| | | DAY 1 | DAY 2 | DAY 3 | DAY 4 | DAY 5 |
| --- | --- | --- | --- | --- | --- | --- |
| FLOW | LIGHT | | | | | |
| | MEDIUM | | | | | |
| | HEAVY | | | | | |
| COLOR | RED | | | | | |
| | PINK | | | | | |
| | RUSTY | | | | | |
| | OTHER | | | | | |

Use this chart to track your period patterns. We encourage you to write directly in the book, but if you'd like to track your period for longer, we suggest you photocopy this page or copy it into a journal or notebook.

| | | DAY 1 | DAY 2 | DAY 3 | DAY 4 | DAY 5 |
|---|---|---|---|---|---|---|
| SYMPTOMS | CRAMPS | | | | | |
| | HEADACHE | | | | | |
| | TENDER BREASTS | | | | | |
| | BLOATING | | | | | |
| | DIARRHEA | | | | | |
| | ACNE | | | | | |
| | OTHER | | | | | |
| EMOTIONS | HAPPY | | | | | |
| | SAD | | | | | |
| | SENSITIVE | | | | | |
| | ANGRY | | | | | |
| | ANXIOUS | | | | | |
| | OTHER | | | | | |
| NOTES | | | | | | |

# Reflections on Month Five:

## WHAT WAS CHALLENGING?
## WHAT IMPROVED?
## WHAT CHANGES DO I WANT TO TRY?

Special thanks to our teacher Victoria Raven Hyndman, who directly inspired some of these chapters. Victoria teaches the wisdom of Ayurveda in an exceptionally beautiful way, which she in turn received from her teacher Dr. Vasant Lad.

Library of Congress Cataloging-in-Publication Data
Names: Blohberger, Julia, author. | Neeter, Roos, author. | Steenbergen, Roel, illustrator.
Title: Good flow : your holistic guide to the best period of your life / Julia Blohberger, and Roos Neeter : illustrations by Roel Steenbergen.
Other titles: Your holistic guide to the best period of your life
Description: Philadelphia : Quirk Books, [2023] | Series: Feel good; 3 | Summary: "A handbook for understanding the connections between menstruation and overall wellness, and for using Ayurvedic principles and lifestyle adjustments to improve the experience of menstruating"— Provided by publisher.
Identifiers: LCCN 2023022189 (print) | LCCN 2023022190 (ebook) | ISBN 9781683693611 (paperback) | ISBN 9781683693628 (ebook)
Subjects: LCSH: Menstruation—Popular works. | Women—Health and hygiene— Popular works. | Medicine, Ayurvedic—Popular works.
Classification: LCC QP263 .B53 2023 (print) | LCC QP263 (ebook) | DDC 612.662— dc23/eng/20230602
LC record available at https://lccn.loc.gov/2023022189
LC ebook record available at https://lccn.loc.gov/2023022190

ISBN: 978-1-68369-361-1

Printed in China

Typeset in Greycliff, Larosa, and Quiche

Designed by Paige Graff
Production management by John J. McGurk

First published in Dutch by Kosmos Uitgevers, The Netherlands in 2023.
Illustrations by Roel Steenbergen.

Quirk Books
215 Church Street
Philadelphia, PA 19106
quirkbooks.com

10 9 8 7 6 5 4 3 2 1